Blood Sugar Log

This Book Belongs to

_____

_____

_____

Contact Details

_____

_____

_____

DEDICATION

This Blood Sugar Log Journal book is dedicated to all the Diabetics out there who are health conscientious and want to track their blood glucose levels and document their findings in the process.

You are my inspiration for producing books and I'm honored to be a part of keeping all of your Blood Sugar notes and records organized.

This journal notebook will help you record your details about your diabetes.

Thoughtfully put together with these sections to record: Date, Daily Readings for Breakfast, Lunch, Dinner & Bedtime, & Notes Section.

HOW TO USE THIS BOOK:

The purpose of this book is to keep all of your Blood Sugar notes all in one place. It will help keep you organized.

This Blood Sugar Log Journal will allow you to accurately document every detail about your blood glucose levels. It's a great way to chart your course through becoming a healthy diabetic.

Here are examples of the prompts for you to fill in and write about your experience in this book:

1. Date - Write the date for the week of.

2. Daily Readings - Record your readings for every day of the week Sunday through Saturday.

3. Breakfast, Lunch, Dinner & Bedtime - Log your readings before and after each meal.

4. Notes Section - Keeping track of any other additional important information you want such as blood pressure readings, food intake diary, monitor insulin used, exercise, snacks, carbs, how well you felt, etc.

Enjoy!

BLOOD SUGAR LOG

Notes _____

_____

_____

_____

WEEK OF: __/__/__	SUNDAY		MONDAY		TUESDAY	
	before	after	before	after	before	after
Breakfast						
Lunch						
Dinner						
Bedtime						

WEEK OF: __/__/__	SUNDAY		MONDAY		TUESDAY	
	before	after	before	after	before	after
Breakfast						
Lunch						
Dinner						
Bedtime						

WEEK OF: __/__/__	SUNDAY		MONDAY		TUESDAY	
	before	after	before	after	before	after
Breakfast						
Lunch						
Dinner						
Bedtime						

WEEK OF: __/__/__	SUNDAY		MONDAY		TUESDAY	
	before	after	before	after	before	after
Breakfast						
Lunch						
Dinner						
Bedtime						

BLOOD SUGAR LOG

Notes _____

_____

_____

_____

WEDNESDAY		THURSDAY		FRIDAY		SATURDAY	
before	after	before	after	before	after	before	after

WEDNESDAY		THURSDAY		FRIDAY		SATURDAY	
before	after	before	after	before	after	before	after

WEDNESDAY		THURSDAY		FRIDAY		SATURDAY	
before	after	before	after	before	after	before	after

WEDNESDAY		THURSDAY		FRIDAY		SATURDAY	
before	after	before	after	before	after	before	after

BLOOD SUGAR LOG

Notes _____

_____

_____

_____

WEEK OF: __/__/__	SUNDAY		MONDAY		TUESDAY	
	before	after	before	after	before	after
Breakfast						
Lunch						
Dinner						
Bedtime						

WEEK OF: __/__/__	SUNDAY		MONDAY		TUESDAY	
	before	after	before	after	before	after
Breakfast						
Lunch						
Dinner						
Bedtime						

WEEK OF: __/__/__	SUNDAY		MONDAY		TUESDAY	
	before	after	before	after	before	after
Breakfast						
Lunch						
Dinner						
Bedtime						

WEEK OF: __/__/__	SUNDAY		MONDAY		TUESDAY	
	before	after	before	after	before	after
Breakfast						
Lunch						
Dinner						
Bedtime						

BLOOD SUGAR LOG

Notes _____

_____

_____

_____

WEDNESDAY		THURSDAY		FRIDAY		SATURDAY	
before	after	before	after	before	after	before	after

WEDNESDAY		THURSDAY		FRIDAY		SATURDAY	
before	after	before	after	before	after	before	after

WEDNESDAY		THURSDAY		FRIDAY		SATURDAY	
before	after	before	after	before	after	before	after

WEDNESDAY		THURSDAY		FRIDAY		SATURDAY	
before	after	before	after	before	after	before	after

BLOOD SUGAR LOG

Notes _____

_____

_____

_____

WEEK OF: __/__/__	SUNDAY		MONDAY		TUESDAY	
	before	after	before	after	before	after
Breakfast						
Lunch						
Dinner						
Bedtime						

WEEK OF: __/__/__	SUNDAY		MONDAY		TUESDAY	
	before	after	before	after	before	after
Breakfast						
Lunch						
Dinner						
Bedtime						

WEEK OF: __/__/__	SUNDAY		MONDAY		TUESDAY	
	before	after	before	after	before	after
Breakfast						
Lunch						
Dinner						
Bedtime						

WEEK OF: __/__/__	SUNDAY		MONDAY		TUESDAY	
	before	after	before	after	before	after
Breakfast						
Lunch						
Dinner						
Bedtime						

BLOOD SUGAR LOG

Notes _____

_____

_____

WEDNESDAY		THURSDAY		FRIDAY		SATURDAY	
before	after	before	after	before	after	before	after

WEDNESDAY		THURSDAY		FRIDAY		SATURDAY	
before	after	before	after	before	after	before	after

WEDNESDAY		THURSDAY		FRIDAY		SATURDAY	
before	after	before	after	before	after	before	after

WEDNESDAY		THURSDAY		FRIDAY		SATURDAY	
before	after	before	after	before	after	before	after

BLOOD SUGAR LOG

Notes _____

_____

_____

_____

WEEK OF: __/__/__	SUNDAY		MONDAY		TUESDAY	
	before	after	before	after	before	after
Breakfast						
Lunch						
Dinner						
Bedtime						

WEEK OF: __/__/__	SUNDAY		MONDAY		TUESDAY	
	before	after	before	after	before	after
Breakfast						
Lunch						
Dinner						
Bedtime						

WEEK OF: __/__/__	SUNDAY		MONDAY		TUESDAY	
	before	after	before	after	before	after
Breakfast						
Lunch						
Dinner						
Bedtime						

WEEK OF: __/__/__	SUNDAY		MONDAY		TUESDAY	
	before	after	before	after	before	after
Breakfast						
Lunch						
Dinner						
Bedtime						

BLOOD SUGAR LOG

Notes _____

_____

_____

_____

WEDNESDAY		THURSDAY		FRIDAY		SATURDAY	
before	after	before	after	before	after	before	after

WEDNESDAY		THURSDAY		FRIDAY		SATURDAY	
before	after	before	after	before	after	before	after

WEDNESDAY		THURSDAY		FRIDAY		SATURDAY	
before	after	before	after	before	after	before	after

WEDNESDAY		THURSDAY		FRIDAY		SATURDAY	
before	after	before	after	before	after	before	after

BLOOD SUGAR LOG

Notes _____

_____

_____

_____

WEEK OF: __/__/__	SUNDAY		MONDAY		TUESDAY	
	before	after	before	after	before	after
Breakfast						
Lunch						
Dinner						
Bedtime						

WEEK OF: __/__/__	SUNDAY		MONDAY		TUESDAY	
	before	after	before	after	before	after
Breakfast						
Lunch						
Dinner						
Bedtime						

WEEK OF: __/__/__	SUNDAY		MONDAY		TUESDAY	
	before	after	before	after	before	after
Breakfast						
Lunch						
Dinner						
Bedtime						

WEEK OF: __/__/__	SUNDAY		MONDAY		TUESDAY	
	before	after	before	after	before	after
Breakfast						
Lunch						
Dinner						
Bedtime						

BLOOD SUGAR LOG

Notes _____

_____

_____

_____

WEDNESDAY		THURSDAY		FRIDAY		SATURDAY	
before	after	before	after	before	after	before	after

WEDNESDAY		THURSDAY		FRIDAY		SATURDAY	
before	after	before	after	before	after	before	after

WEDNESDAY		THURSDAY		FRIDAY		SATURDAY	
before	after	before	after	before	after	before	after

WEDNESDAY		THURSDAY		FRIDAY		SATURDAY	
before	after	before	after	before	after	before	after

BLOOD SUGAR LOG

Notes
_____

WEEK OF: __/__/__	SUNDAY		MONDAY		TUESDAY	
	before	after	before	after	before	after
Breakfast						
Lunch						
Dinner						
Bedtime						

WEEK OF: __/__/__	SUNDAY		MONDAY		TUESDAY	
	before	after	before	after	before	after
Breakfast						
Lunch						
Dinner						
Bedtime						

WEEK OF: __/__/__	SUNDAY		MONDAY		TUESDAY	
	before	after	before	after	before	after
Breakfast						
Lunch						
Dinner						
Bedtime						

WEEK OF: __/__/__	SUNDAY		MONDAY		TUESDAY	
	before	after	before	after	before	after
Breakfast						
Lunch						
Dinner						
Bedtime						

BLOOD SUGAR LOG

Notes

_____

_____

_____

_____

WEDNESDAY		THURSDAY		FRIDAY		SATURDAY	
before	after	before	after	before	after	before	after

WEDNESDAY		THURSDAY		FRIDAY		SATURDAY	
before	after	before	after	before	after	before	after

WEDNESDAY		THURSDAY		FRIDAY		SATURDAY	
before	after	before	after	before	after	before	after

WEDNESDAY		THURSDAY		FRIDAY		SATURDAY	
before	after	before	after	before	after	before	after

BLOOD SUGAR LOG

Notes _____

_____

_____

WEEK OF: __/__/__	SUNDAY		MONDAY		TUESDAY	
	before	after	before	after	before	after
Breakfast						
Lunch						
Dinner						
Bedtime						

WEEK OF: __/__/__	SUNDAY		MONDAY		TUESDAY	
	before	after	before	after	before	after
Breakfast						
Lunch						
Dinner						
Bedtime						

WEEK OF: __/__/__	SUNDAY		MONDAY		TUESDAY	
	before	after	before	after	before	after
Breakfast						
Lunch						
Dinner						
Bedtime						

WEEK OF: __/__/__	SUNDAY		MONDAY		TUESDAY	
	before	after	before	after	before	after
Breakfast						
Lunch						
Dinner						
Bedtime						

BLOOD SUGAR LOG

Notes _____

_____

_____

_____

WEDNESDAY		THURSDAY		FRIDAY		SATURDAY	
before	after	before	after	before	after	before	after

WEDNESDAY		THURSDAY		FRIDAY		SATURDAY	
before	after	before	after	before	after	before	after

WEDNESDAY		THURSDAY		FRIDAY		SATURDAY	
before	after	before	after	before	after	before	after

WEDNESDAY		THURSDAY		FRIDAY		SATURDAY	
before	after	before	after	before	after	before	after

BLOOD SUGAR LOG

Notes _____

_____

_____

_____

WEEK OF: __/__/__	SUNDAY		MONDAY		TUESDAY	
	before	after	before	after	before	after
Breakfast						
Lunch						
Dinner						
Bedtime						

WEEK OF: __/__/__	SUNDAY		MONDAY		TUESDAY	
	before	after	before	after	before	after
Breakfast						
Lunch						
Dinner						
Bedtime						

WEEK OF: __/__/__	SUNDAY		MONDAY		TUESDAY	
	before	after	before	after	before	after
Breakfast						
Lunch						
Dinner						
Bedtime						

WEEK OF: __/__/__	SUNDAY		MONDAY		TUESDAY	
	before	after	before	after	before	after
Breakfast						
Lunch						
Dinner						
Bedtime						

BLOOD SUGAR LOG

Notes _____

_____

_____

WEDNESDAY		THURSDAY		FRIDAY		SATURDAY	
before	after	before	after	before	after	before	after

WEDNESDAY		THURSDAY		FRIDAY		SATURDAY	
before	after	before	after	before	after	before	after

WEDNESDAY		THURSDAY		FRIDAY		SATURDAY	
before	after	before	after	before	after	before	after

WEDNESDAY		THURSDAY		FRIDAY		SATURDAY	
before	after	before	after	before	after	before	after

BLOOD SUGAR LOG

Notes _____

_____

_____

_____

WEEK OF: __/__/__	SUNDAY		MONDAY		TUESDAY	
	before	after	before	after	before	after
Breakfast						
Lunch						
Dinner						
Bedtime						

WEEK OF: __/__/__	SUNDAY		MONDAY		TUESDAY	
	before	after	before	after	before	after
Breakfast						
Lunch						
Dinner						
Bedtime						

WEEK OF: __/__/__	SUNDAY		MONDAY		TUESDAY	
	before	after	before	after	before	after
Breakfast						
Lunch						
Dinner						
Bedtime						

WEEK OF: __/__/__	SUNDAY		MONDAY		TUESDAY	
	before	after	before	after	before	after
Breakfast						
Lunch						
Dinner						
Bedtime						

BLOOD SUGAR LOG

Notes _____

_____

_____

_____

WEDNESDAY		THURSDAY		FRIDAY		SATURDAY	
before	after	before	after	before	after	before	after

WEDNESDAY		THURSDAY		FRIDAY		SATURDAY	
before	after	before	after	before	after	before	after

WEDNESDAY		THURSDAY		FRIDAY		SATURDAY	
before	after	before	after	before	after	before	after

WEDNESDAY		THURSDAY		FRIDAY		SATURDAY	
before	after	before	after	before	after	before	after

BLOOD SUGAR LOG

Notes _____

_____

_____

WEEK OF: __/__/__	SUNDAY		MONDAY		TUESDAY	
	before	after	before	after	before	after
Breakfast						
Lunch						
Dinner						
Bedtime						

WEEK OF: __/__/__	SUNDAY		MONDAY		TUESDAY	
	before	after	before	after	before	after
Breakfast						
Lunch						
Dinner						
Bedtime						

WEEK OF: __/__/__	SUNDAY		MONDAY		TUESDAY	
	before	after	before	after	before	after
Breakfast						
Lunch						
Dinner						
Bedtime						

WEEK OF: __/__/__	SUNDAY		MONDAY		TUESDAY	
	before	after	before	after	before	after
Breakfast						
Lunch						
Dinner						
Bedtime						

BLOOD SUGAR LOG

Notes _____

_____

_____

_____

WEDNESDAY		THURSDAY		FRIDAY		SATURDAY	
before	after	before	after	before	after	before	after

WEDNESDAY		THURSDAY		FRIDAY		SATURDAY	
before	after	before	after	before	after	before	after

WEDNESDAY		THURSDAY		FRIDAY		SATURDAY	
before	after	before	after	before	after	before	after

WEDNESDAY		THURSDAY		FRIDAY		SATURDAY	
before	after	before	after	before	after	before	after

BLOOD SUGAR LOG

Notes _____

_____

_____

_____

WEEK OF: __/__/__	SUNDAY		MONDAY		TUESDAY	
	before	after	before	after	before	after
Breakfast						
Lunch						
Dinner						
Bedtime						

WEEK OF: __/__/__	SUNDAY		MONDAY		TUESDAY	
	before	after	before	after	before	after
Breakfast						
Lunch						
Dinner						
Bedtime						

WEEK OF: __/__/__	SUNDAY		MONDAY		TUESDAY	
	before	after	before	after	before	after
Breakfast						
Lunch						
Dinner						
Bedtime						

WEEK OF: __/__/__	SUNDAY		MONDAY		TUESDAY	
	before	after	before	after	before	after
Breakfast						
Lunch						
Dinner						
Bedtime						

BLOOD SUGAR LOG

Notes _____

_____

_____

_____

WEDNESDAY		THURSDAY		FRIDAY		SATURDAY	
before	after	before	after	before	after	before	after

WEDNESDAY		THURSDAY		FRIDAY		SATURDAY	
before	after	before	after	before	after	before	after

WEDNESDAY		THURSDAY		FRIDAY		SATURDAY	
before	after	before	after	before	after	before	after

WEDNESDAY		THURSDAY		FRIDAY		SATURDAY	
before	after	before	after	before	after	before	after

BLOOD SUGAR LOG

Notes _____

_____

_____

_____

WEEK OF: __/__/__	SUNDAY		MONDAY		TUESDAY	
	before	after	before	after	before	after
Breakfast						
Lunch						
Dinner						
Bedtime						

WEEK OF: __/__/__	SUNDAY		MONDAY		TUESDAY	
	before	after	before	after	before	after
Breakfast						
Lunch						
Dinner						
Bedtime						

WEEK OF: __/__/__	SUNDAY		MONDAY		TUESDAY	
	before	after	before	after	before	after
Breakfast						
Lunch						
Dinner						
Bedtime						

WEEK OF: __/__/__	SUNDAY		MONDAY		TUESDAY	
	before	after	before	after	before	after
Breakfast						
Lunch						
Dinner						
Bedtime						

BLOOD SUGAR LOG

Notes

WEDNESDAY		THURSDAY		FRIDAY		SATURDAY	
before	after	before	after	before	after	before	after

WEDNESDAY		THURSDAY		FRIDAY		SATURDAY	
before	after	before	after	before	after	before	after

WEDNESDAY		THURSDAY		FRIDAY		SATURDAY	
before	after	before	after	before	after	before	after

WEDNESDAY		THURSDAY		FRIDAY		SATURDAY	
before	after	before	after	before	after	before	after

BLOOD SUGAR LOG

Notes

_____

_____

_____

WEEK OF: __/__/__	SUNDAY		MONDAY		TUESDAY	
	before	after	before	after	before	after
Breakfast						
Lunch						
Dinner						
Bedtime						

WEEK OF: __/__/__	SUNDAY		MONDAY		TUESDAY	
	before	after	before	after	before	after
Breakfast						
Lunch						
Dinner						
Bedtime						

WEEK OF: __/__/__	SUNDAY		MONDAY		TUESDAY	
	before	after	before	after	before	after
Breakfast						
Lunch						
Dinner						
Bedtime						

WEEK OF: __/__/__	SUNDAY		MONDAY		TUESDAY	
	before	after	before	after	before	after
Breakfast						
Lunch						
Dinner						
Bedtime						

BLOOD SUGAR LOG

Notes
_____
_____
_____
_____

WEDNESDAY		THURSDAY		FRIDAY		SATURDAY	
before	after	before	after	before	after	before	after

WEDNESDAY		THURSDAY		FRIDAY		SATURDAY	
before	after	before	after	before	after	before	after

WEDNESDAY		THURSDAY		FRIDAY		SATURDAY	
before	after	before	after	before	after	before	after

WEDNESDAY		THURSDAY		FRIDAY		SATURDAY	
before	after	before	after	before	after	before	after

BLOOD SUGAR LOG

Notes _____

WEEK OF: __/__/__	SUNDAY		MONDAY		TUESDAY	
	before	after	before	after	before	after
Breakfast						
Lunch						
Dinner						
Bedtime						

WEEK OF: __/__/__	SUNDAY		MONDAY		TUESDAY	
	before	after	before	after	before	after
Breakfast						
Lunch						
Dinner						
Bedtime						

WEEK OF: __/__/__	SUNDAY		MONDAY		TUESDAY	
	before	after	before	after	before	after
Breakfast						
Lunch						
Dinner						
Bedtime						

WEEK OF: __/__/__	SUNDAY		MONDAY		TUESDAY	
	before	after	before	after	before	after
Breakfast						
Lunch						
Dinner						
Bedtime						

BLOOD SUGAR LOG

Notes _____

_____

_____

_____

WEDNESDAY		THURSDAY		FRIDAY		SATURDAY	
before	after	before	after	before	after	before	after

WEDNESDAY		THURSDAY		FRIDAY		SATURDAY	
before	after	before	after	before	after	before	after

WEDNESDAY		THURSDAY		FRIDAY		SATURDAY	
before	after	before	after	before	after	before	after

WEDNESDAY		THURSDAY		FRIDAY		SATURDAY	
before	after	before	after	before	after	before	after

BLOOD SUGAR LOG

Notes _____

_____

_____

_____

WEEK OF: __/__/__	SUNDAY		MONDAY		TUESDAY	
	before	after	before	after	before	after
Breakfast						
Lunch						
Dinner						
Bedtime						

WEEK OF: __/__/__	SUNDAY		MONDAY		TUESDAY	
	before	after	before	after	before	after
Breakfast						
Lunch						
Dinner						
Bedtime						

WEEK OF: __/__/__	SUNDAY		MONDAY		TUESDAY	
	before	after	before	after	before	after
Breakfast						
Lunch						
Dinner						
Bedtime						

WEEK OF: __/__/__	SUNDAY		MONDAY		TUESDAY	
	before	after	before	after	before	after
Breakfast						
Lunch						
Dinner						
Bedtime						

BLOOD SUGAR LOG

Notes

WEDNESDAY		THURSDAY		FRIDAY		SATURDAY	
before	after	before	after	before	after	before	after

WEDNESDAY		THURSDAY		FRIDAY		SATURDAY	
before	after	before	after	before	after	before	after

WEDNESDAY		THURSDAY		FRIDAY		SATURDAY	
before	after	before	after	before	after	before	after

WEDNESDAY		THURSDAY		FRIDAY		SATURDAY	
before	after	before	after	before	after	before	after

BLOOD SUGAR LOG

Notes
_____

WEEK OF: __/__/__	SUNDAY		MONDAY		TUESDAY	
	before	after	before	after	before	after
Breakfast						
Lunch						
Dinner						
Bedtime						

WEEK OF: __/__/__	SUNDAY		MONDAY		TUESDAY	
	before	after	before	after	before	after
Breakfast						
Lunch						
Dinner						
Bedtime						

WEEK OF: __/__/__	SUNDAY		MONDAY		TUESDAY	
	before	after	before	after	before	after
Breakfast						
Lunch						
Dinner						
Bedtime						

WEEK OF: __/__/__	SUNDAY		MONDAY		TUESDAY	
	before	after	before	after	before	after
Breakfast						
Lunch						
Dinner						
Bedtime						

BLOOD SUGAR LOG

Notes _____

_____

_____

_____

WEDNESDAY		THURSDAY		FRIDAY		SATURDAY	
before	after	before	after	before	after	before	after

WEDNESDAY		THURSDAY		FRIDAY		SATURDAY	
before	after	before	after	before	after	before	after

WEDNESDAY		THURSDAY		FRIDAY		SATURDAY	
before	after	before	after	before	after	before	after

WEDNESDAY		THURSDAY		FRIDAY		SATURDAY	
before	after	before	after	before	after	before	after

BLOOD SUGAR LOG

Notes _____

_____

_____

_____

WEEK OF: __/__/__	SUNDAY		MONDAY		TUESDAY	
	before	after	before	after	before	after
Breakfast						
Lunch						
Dinner						
Bedtime						

WEEK OF: __/__/__	SUNDAY		MONDAY		TUESDAY	
	before	after	before	after	before	after
Breakfast						
Lunch						
Dinner						
Bedtime						

WEEK OF: __/__/__	SUNDAY		MONDAY		TUESDAY	
	before	after	before	after	before	after
Breakfast						
Lunch						
Dinner						
Bedtime						

WEEK OF: __/__/__	SUNDAY		MONDAY		TUESDAY	
	before	after	before	after	before	after
Breakfast						
Lunch						
Dinner						
Bedtime						

BLOOD SUGAR LOG

Notes _____

_____

_____

_____

WEDNESDAY		THURSDAY		FRIDAY		SATURDAY	
before	after	before	after	before	after	before	after

WEDNESDAY		THURSDAY		FRIDAY		SATURDAY	
before	after	before	after	before	after	before	after

WEDNESDAY		THURSDAY		FRIDAY		SATURDAY	
before	after	before	after	before	after	before	after

WEDNESDAY		THURSDAY		FRIDAY		SATURDAY	
before	after	before	after	before	after	before	after

BLOOD SUGAR LOG

Notes _____

_____

_____

_____

WEEK OF: __/__/__	SUNDAY		MONDAY		TUESDAY	
	before	after	before	after	before	after
Breakfast						
Lunch						
Dinner						
Bedtime						

WEEK OF: __/__/__	SUNDAY		MONDAY		TUESDAY	
	before	after	before	after	before	after
Breakfast						
Lunch						
Dinner						
Bedtime						

WEEK OF: __/__/__	SUNDAY		MONDAY		TUESDAY	
	before	after	before	after	before	after
Breakfast						
Lunch						
Dinner						
Bedtime						

WEEK OF: __/__/__	SUNDAY		MONDAY		TUESDAY	
	before	after	before	after	before	after
Breakfast						
Lunch						
Dinner						
Bedtime						

BLOOD SUGAR LOG

Notes
_____
_____
_____
_____

WEDNESDAY		THURSDAY		FRIDAY		SATURDAY	
before	after	before	after	before	after	before	after

WEDNESDAY		THURSDAY		FRIDAY		SATURDAY	
before	after	before	after	before	after	before	after

WEDNESDAY		THURSDAY		FRIDAY		SATURDAY	
before	after	before	after	before	after	before	after

WEDNESDAY		THURSDAY		FRIDAY		SATURDAY	
before	after	before	after	before	after	before	after

BLOOD SUGAR LOG

Notes _____
_____
_____
_____

WEEK OF: __/__/__	SUNDAY		MONDAY		TUESDAY	
	before	after	before	after	before	after
Breakfast						
Lunch						
Dinner						
Bedtime						

WEEK OF: __/__/__	SUNDAY		MONDAY		TUESDAY	
	before	after	before	after	before	after
Breakfast						
Lunch						
Dinner						
Bedtime						

WEEK OF: __/__/__	SUNDAY		MONDAY		TUESDAY	
	before	after	before	after	before	after
Breakfast						
Lunch						
Dinner						
Bedtime						

WEEK OF: __/__/__	SUNDAY		MONDAY		TUESDAY	
	before	after	before	after	before	after
Breakfast						
Lunch						
Dinner						
Bedtime						

BLOOD SUGAR LOG

Notes

WEDNESDAY		THURSDAY		FRIDAY		SATURDAY	
before	after	before	after	before	after	before	after

WEDNESDAY		THURSDAY		FRIDAY		SATURDAY	
before	after	before	after	before	after	before	after

WEDNESDAY		THURSDAY		FRIDAY		SATURDAY	
before	after	before	after	before	after	before	after

WEDNESDAY		THURSDAY		FRIDAY		SATURDAY	
before	after	before	after	before	after	before	after

BLOOD SUGAR LOG

Notes _____

_____

_____

_____

WEEK OF: __/__/__	SUNDAY		MONDAY		TUESDAY	
	before	after	before	after	before	after
Breakfast						
Lunch						
Dinner						
Bedtime						

WEEK OF: __/__/__	SUNDAY		MONDAY		TUESDAY	
	before	after	before	after	before	after
Breakfast						
Lunch						
Dinner						
Bedtime						

WEEK OF: __/__/__	SUNDAY		MONDAY		TUESDAY	
	before	after	before	after	before	after
Breakfast						
Lunch						
Dinner						
Bedtime						

WEEK OF: __/__/__	SUNDAY		MONDAY		TUESDAY	
	before	after	before	after	before	after
Breakfast						
Lunch						
Dinner						
Bedtime						

BLOOD SUGAR LOG

Notes

WEDNESDAY		THURSDAY		FRIDAY		SATURDAY	
before	after	before	after	before	after	before	after

WEDNESDAY		THURSDAY		FRIDAY		SATURDAY	
before	after	before	after	before	after	before	after

WEDNESDAY		THURSDAY		FRIDAY		SATURDAY	
before	after	before	after	before	after	before	after

WEDNESDAY		THURSDAY		FRIDAY		SATURDAY	
before	after	before	after	before	after	before	after

BLOOD SUGAR LOG

Notes _____
_____
_____
_____

WEEK OF: __/__/__	SUNDAY		MONDAY		TUESDAY	
	before	after	before	after	before	after
Breakfast						
Lunch						
Dinner						
Bedtime						

WEEK OF: __/__/__	SUNDAY		MONDAY		TUESDAY	
	before	after	before	after	before	after
Breakfast						
Lunch						
Dinner						
Bedtime						

WEEK OF: __/__/__	SUNDAY		MONDAY		TUESDAY	
	before	after	before	after	before	after
Breakfast						
Lunch						
Dinner						
Bedtime						

WEEK OF: __/__/__	SUNDAY		MONDAY		TUESDAY	
	before	after	before	after	before	after
Breakfast						
Lunch						
Dinner						
Bedtime						

BLOOD SUGAR LOG

Notes _____

_____

_____

_____

WEDNESDAY		THURSDAY		FRIDAY		SATURDAY	
before	after	before	after	before	after	before	after

WEDNESDAY		THURSDAY		FRIDAY		SATURDAY	
before	after	before	after	before	after	before	after

WEDNESDAY		THURSDAY		FRIDAY		SATURDAY	
before	after	before	after	before	after	before	after

WEDNESDAY		THURSDAY		FRIDAY		SATURDAY	
before	after	before	after	before	after	before	after

BLOOD SUGAR LOG

Notes _____

_____

_____

_____

WEEK OF: __/__/__	SUNDAY		MONDAY		TUESDAY	
	before	after	before	after	before	after
Breakfast						
Lunch						
Dinner						
Bedtime						

WEEK OF: __/__/__	SUNDAY		MONDAY		TUESDAY	
	before	after	before	after	before	after
Breakfast						
Lunch						
Dinner						
Bedtime						

WEEK OF: __/__/__	SUNDAY		MONDAY		TUESDAY	
	before	after	before	after	before	after
Breakfast						
Lunch						
Dinner						
Bedtime						

WEEK OF: __/__/__	SUNDAY		MONDAY		TUESDAY	
	before	after	before	after	before	after
Breakfast						
Lunch						
Dinner						
Bedtime						

BLOOD SUGAR LOG

Notes
_____
_____
_____
_____

WEDNESDAY		THURSDAY		FRIDAY		SATURDAY	
before	after	before	after	before	after	before	after

WEDNESDAY		THURSDAY		FRIDAY		SATURDAY	
before	after	before	after	before	after	before	after

WEDNESDAY		THURSDAY		FRIDAY		SATURDAY	
before	after	before	after	before	after	before	after

WEDNESDAY		THURSDAY		FRIDAY		SATURDAY	
before	after	before	after	before	after	before	after

BLOOD SUGAR LOG

Notes _____
_____
_____
_____

WEEK OF: __/__/__	SUNDAY		MONDAY		TUESDAY	
	before	after	before	after	before	after
Breakfast						
Lunch						
Dinner						
Bedtime						

WEEK OF: __/__/__	SUNDAY		MONDAY		TUESDAY	
	before	after	before	after	before	after
Breakfast						
Lunch						
Dinner						
Bedtime						

WEEK OF: __/__/__	SUNDAY		MONDAY		TUESDAY	
	before	after	before	after	before	after
Breakfast						
Lunch						
Dinner						
Bedtime						

WEEK OF: __/__/__	SUNDAY		MONDAY		TUESDAY	
	before	after	before	after	before	after
Breakfast						
Lunch						
Dinner						
Bedtime						

BLOOD SUGAR LOG

Notes _____

_____

_____

WEDNESDAY		THURSDAY		FRIDAY		SATURDAY	
before	after	before	after	before	after	before	after

WEDNESDAY		THURSDAY		FRIDAY		SATURDAY	
before	after	before	after	before	after	before	after

WEDNESDAY		THURSDAY		FRIDAY		SATURDAY	
before	after	before	after	before	after	before	after

WEDNESDAY		THURSDAY		FRIDAY		SATURDAY	
before	after	before	after	before	after	before	after

BLOOD SUGAR LOG

Notes _____

_____

_____

_____

WEEK OF: __/__/__	SUNDAY		MONDAY		TUESDAY	
	before	after	before	after	before	after
Breakfast						
Lunch						
Dinner						
Bedtime						

WEEK OF: __/__/__	SUNDAY		MONDAY		TUESDAY	
	before	after	before	after	before	after
Breakfast						
Lunch						
Dinner						
Bedtime						

WEEK OF: __/__/__	SUNDAY		MONDAY		TUESDAY	
	before	after	before	after	before	after
Breakfast						
Lunch						
Dinner						
Bedtime						

WEEK OF: __/__/__	SUNDAY		MONDAY		TUESDAY	
	before	after	before	after	before	after
Breakfast						
Lunch						
Dinner						
Bedtime						

BLOOD SUGAR LOG

Notes _____

_____

_____

_____

WEDNESDAY		THURSDAY		FRIDAY		SATURDAY	
before	after	before	after	before	after	before	after

WEDNESDAY		THURSDAY		FRIDAY		SATURDAY	
before	after	before	after	before	after	before	after

WEDNESDAY		THURSDAY		FRIDAY		SATURDAY	
before	after	before	after	before	after	before	after

WEDNESDAY		THURSDAY		FRIDAY		SATURDAY	
before	after	before	after	before	after	before	after

BLOOD SUGAR LOG

Notes _____

_____

_____

_____

WEEK OF: __/__/__	SUNDAY		MONDAY		TUESDAY	
	before	after	before	after	before	after
Breakfast						
Lunch						
Dinner						
Bedtime						

WEEK OF: __/__/__	SUNDAY		MONDAY		TUESDAY	
	before	after	before	after	before	after
Breakfast						
Lunch						
Dinner						
Bedtime						

WEEK OF: __/__/__	SUNDAY		MONDAY		TUESDAY	
	before	after	before	after	before	after
Breakfast						
Lunch						
Dinner						
Bedtime						

WEEK OF: __/__/__	SUNDAY		MONDAY		TUESDAY	
	before	after	before	after	before	after
Breakfast						
Lunch						
Dinner						
Bedtime						

BLOOD SUGAR LOG

Notes

WEDNESDAY		THURSDAY		FRIDAY		SATURDAY	
before	after	before	after	before	after	before	after

WEDNESDAY		THURSDAY		FRIDAY		SATURDAY	
before	after	before	after	before	after	before	after

WEDNESDAY		THURSDAY		FRIDAY		SATURDAY	
before	after	before	after	before	after	before	after

WEDNESDAY		THURSDAY		FRIDAY		SATURDAY	
before	after	before	after	before	after	before	after

BLOOD SUGAR LOG

Notes _____
_____
_____
_____

WEEK OF: __/__/__	SUNDAY		MONDAY		TUESDAY	
	before	after	before	after	before	after
Breakfast						
Lunch						
Dinner						
Bedtime						

WEEK OF: __/__/__	SUNDAY		MONDAY		TUESDAY	
	before	after	before	after	before	after
Breakfast						
Lunch						
Dinner						
Bedtime						

WEEK OF: __/__/__	SUNDAY		MONDAY		TUESDAY	
	before	after	before	after	before	after
Breakfast						
Lunch						
Dinner						
Bedtime						

WEEK OF: __/__/__	SUNDAY		MONDAY		TUESDAY	
	before	after	before	after	before	after
Breakfast						
Lunch						
Dinner						
Bedtime						

BLOOD SUGAR LOG

Notes

WEDNESDAY		THURSDAY		FRIDAY		SATURDAY	
before	after	before	after	before	after	before	after

WEDNESDAY		THURSDAY		FRIDAY		SATURDAY	
before	after	before	after	before	after	before	after

WEDNESDAY		THURSDAY		FRIDAY		SATURDAY	
before	after	before	after	before	after	before	after

WEDNESDAY		THURSDAY		FRIDAY		SATURDAY	
before	after	before	after	before	after	before	after

BLOOD SUGAR LOG

Notes _____
_____
_____
_____

WEEK OF: __/__/__	SUNDAY		MONDAY		TUESDAY	
	before	after	before	after	before	after
Breakfast						
Lunch						
Dinner						
Bedtime						

WEEK OF: __/__/__	SUNDAY		MONDAY		TUESDAY	
	before	after	before	after	before	after
Breakfast						
Lunch						
Dinner						
Bedtime						

WEEK OF: __/__/__	SUNDAY		MONDAY		TUESDAY	
	before	after	before	after	before	after
Breakfast						
Lunch						
Dinner						
Bedtime						

WEEK OF: __/__/__	SUNDAY		MONDAY		TUESDAY	
	before	after	before	after	before	after
Breakfast						
Lunch						
Dinner						
Bedtime						

BLOOD SUGAR LOG

Notes _____

_____

_____

_____

WEDNESDAY		THURSDAY		FRIDAY		SATURDAY	
before	after	before	after	before	after	before	after

WEDNESDAY		THURSDAY		FRIDAY		SATURDAY	
before	after	before	after	before	after	before	after

WEDNESDAY		THURSDAY		FRIDAY		SATURDAY	
before	after	before	after	before	after	before	after

WEDNESDAY		THURSDAY		FRIDAY		SATURDAY	
before	after	before	after	before	after	before	after

BLOOD SUGAR LOG

Notes _____

_____

_____

_____

WEEK OF: __/__/__	SUNDAY		MONDAY		TUESDAY	
	before	after	before	after	before	after
Breakfast						
Lunch						
Dinner						
Bedtime						

WEEK OF: __/__/__	SUNDAY		MONDAY		TUESDAY	
	before	after	before	after	before	after
Breakfast						
Lunch						
Dinner						
Bedtime						

WEEK OF: __/__/__	SUNDAY		MONDAY		TUESDAY	
	before	after	before	after	before	after
Breakfast						
Lunch						
Dinner						
Bedtime						

WEEK OF: __/__/__	SUNDAY		MONDAY		TUESDAY	
	before	after	before	after	before	after
Breakfast						
Lunch						
Dinner						
Bedtime						

BLOOD SUGAR LOG

Notes _____

_____

_____

_____

WEDNESDAY		THURSDAY		FRIDAY		SATURDAY	
before	after	before	after	before	after	before	after

WEDNESDAY		THURSDAY		FRIDAY		SATURDAY	
before	after	before	after	before	after	before	after

WEDNESDAY		THURSDAY		FRIDAY		SATURDAY	
before	after	before	after	before	after	before	after

WEDNESDAY		THURSDAY		FRIDAY		SATURDAY	
before	after	before	after	before	after	before	after

BLOOD SUGAR LOG

Notes _____
_____
_____
_____

WEEK OF: __/__/__	SUNDAY		MONDAY		TUESDAY	
	before	after	before	after	before	after
Breakfast						
Lunch						
Dinner						
Bedtime						

WEEK OF: __/__/__	SUNDAY		MONDAY		TUESDAY	
	before	after	before	after	before	after
Breakfast						
Lunch						
Dinner						
Bedtime						

WEEK OF: __/__/__	SUNDAY		MONDAY		TUESDAY	
	before	after	before	after	before	after
Breakfast						
Lunch						
Dinner						
Bedtime						

WEEK OF: __/__/__	SUNDAY		MONDAY		TUESDAY	
	before	after	before	after	before	after
Breakfast						
Lunch						
Dinner						
Bedtime						

BLOOD SUGAR LOG

Notes _____

_____

_____

WEDNESDAY		THURSDAY		FRIDAY		SATURDAY	
before	after	before	after	before	after	before	after

WEDNESDAY		THURSDAY		FRIDAY		SATURDAY	
before	after	before	after	before	after	before	after

WEDNESDAY		THURSDAY		FRIDAY		SATURDAY	
before	after	before	after	before	after	before	after

WEDNESDAY		THURSDAY		FRIDAY		SATURDAY	
before	after	before	after	before	after	before	after

BLOOD SUGAR LOG

Notes _____

_____

_____

_____

WEEK OF: __/__/__	SUNDAY		MONDAY		TUESDAY	
	before	after	before	after	before	after
Breakfast						
Lunch						
Dinner						
Bedtime						

WEEK OF: __/__/__	SUNDAY		MONDAY		TUESDAY	
	before	after	before	after	before	after
Breakfast						
Lunch						
Dinner						
Bedtime						

WEEK OF: __/__/__	SUNDAY		MONDAY		TUESDAY	
	before	after	before	after	before	after
Breakfast						
Lunch						
Dinner						
Bedtime						

WEEK OF: __/__/__	SUNDAY		MONDAY		TUESDAY	
	before	after	before	after	before	after
Breakfast						
Lunch						
Dinner						
Bedtime						

BLOOD SUGAR LOG

Notes

WEDNESDAY		THURSDAY		FRIDAY		SATURDAY	
before	after	before	after	before	after	before	after

WEDNESDAY		THURSDAY		FRIDAY		SATURDAY	
before	after	before	after	before	after	before	after

WEDNESDAY		THURSDAY		FRIDAY		SATURDAY	
before	after	before	after	before	after	before	after

WEDNESDAY		THURSDAY		FRIDAY		SATURDAY	
before	after	before	after	before	after	before	after

BLOOD SUGAR LOG

Notes _____

_____

_____

_____

WEEK OF: __/__/__	SUNDAY		MONDAY		TUESDAY	
	before	after	before	after	before	after
Breakfast						
Lunch						
Dinner						
Bedtime						

WEEK OF: __/__/__	SUNDAY		MONDAY		TUESDAY	
	before	after	before	after	before	after
Breakfast						
Lunch						
Dinner						
Bedtime						

WEEK OF: __/__/__	SUNDAY		MONDAY		TUESDAY	
	before	after	before	after	before	after
Breakfast						
Lunch						
Dinner						
Bedtime						

WEEK OF: __/__/__	SUNDAY		MONDAY		TUESDAY	
	before	after	before	after	before	after
Breakfast						
Lunch						
Dinner						
Bedtime						

BLOOD SUGAR LOG

Notes _____

_____

_____

_____

WEDNESDAY		THURSDAY		FRIDAY		SATURDAY	
before	after	before	after	before	after	before	after

WEDNESDAY		THURSDAY		FRIDAY		SATURDAY	
before	after	before	after	before	after	before	after

WEDNESDAY		THURSDAY		FRIDAY		SATURDAY	
before	after	before	after	before	after	before	after

WEDNESDAY		THURSDAY		FRIDAY		SATURDAY	
before	after	before	after	before	after	before	after

BLOOD SUGAR LOG

Notes _____

_____

_____

_____

WEEK OF: __/__/__	SUNDAY		MONDAY		TUESDAY	
	before	after	before	after	before	after
Breakfast						
Lunch						
Dinner						
Bedtime						

WEEK OF: __/__/__	SUNDAY		MONDAY		TUESDAY	
	before	after	before	after	before	after
Breakfast						
Lunch						
Dinner						
Bedtime						

WEEK OF: __/__/__	SUNDAY		MONDAY		TUESDAY	
	before	after	before	after	before	after
Breakfast						
Lunch						
Dinner						
Bedtime						

WEEK OF: __/__/__	SUNDAY		MONDAY		TUESDAY	
	before	after	before	after	before	after
Breakfast						
Lunch						
Dinner						
Bedtime						

BLOOD SUGAR LOG

Notes _____

_____

_____

_____

WEDNESDAY		THURSDAY		FRIDAY		SATURDAY	
before	after	before	after	before	after	before	after

WEDNESDAY		THURSDAY		FRIDAY		SATURDAY	
before	after	before	after	before	after	before	after

WEDNESDAY		THURSDAY		FRIDAY		SATURDAY	
before	after	before	after	before	after	before	after

WEDNESDAY		THURSDAY		FRIDAY		SATURDAY	
before	after	before	after	before	after	before	after

BLOOD SUGAR LOG

Notes _____

_____

_____

_____

WEEK OF: __/__/__	SUNDAY		MONDAY		TUESDAY	
	before	after	before	after	before	after
Breakfast						
Lunch						
Dinner						
Bedtime						

WEEK OF: __/__/__	SUNDAY		MONDAY		TUESDAY	
	before	after	before	after	before	after
Breakfast						
Lunch						
Dinner						
Bedtime						

WEEK OF: __/__/__	SUNDAY		MONDAY		TUESDAY	
	before	after	before	after	before	after
Breakfast						
Lunch						
Dinner						
Bedtime						

WEEK OF: __/__/__	SUNDAY		MONDAY		TUESDAY	
	before	after	before	after	before	after
Breakfast						
Lunch						
Dinner						
Bedtime						

BLOOD SUGAR LOG

Notes _____

_____

_____

_____

WEDNESDAY		THURSDAY		FRIDAY		SATURDAY	
before	after	before	after	before	after	before	after

WEDNESDAY		THURSDAY		FRIDAY		SATURDAY	
before	after	before	after	before	after	before	after

WEDNESDAY		THURSDAY		FRIDAY		SATURDAY	
before	after	before	after	before	after	before	after

WEDNESDAY		THURSDAY		FRIDAY		SATURDAY	
before	after	before	after	before	after	before	after

BLOOD SUGAR LOG

Notes
_____
_____
_____
_____

WEEK OF: __/__/__	SUNDAY		MONDAY		TUESDAY	
	before	after	before	after	before	after
Breakfast						
Lunch						
Dinner						
Bedtime						

WEEK OF: __/__/__	SUNDAY		MONDAY		TUESDAY	
	before	after	before	after	before	after
Breakfast						
Lunch						
Dinner						
Bedtime						

WEEK OF: __/__/__	SUNDAY		MONDAY		TUESDAY	
	before	after	before	after	before	after
Breakfast						
Lunch						
Dinner						
Bedtime						

WEEK OF: __/__/__	SUNDAY		MONDAY		TUESDAY	
	before	after	before	after	before	after
Breakfast						
Lunch						
Dinner						
Bedtime						

BLOOD SUGAR LOG

Notes _____

_____

_____

_____

WEDNESDAY		THURSDAY		FRIDAY		SATURDAY	
before	after	before	after	before	after	before	after

WEDNESDAY		THURSDAY		FRIDAY		SATURDAY	
before	after	before	after	before	after	before	after

WEDNESDAY		THURSDAY		FRIDAY		SATURDAY	
before	after	before	after	before	after	before	after

WEDNESDAY		THURSDAY		FRIDAY		SATURDAY	
before	after	before	after	before	after	before	after

BLOOD SUGAR LOG

Notes _____

_____

_____

_____

WEEK OF: __/__/__	SUNDAY		MONDAY		TUESDAY	
	before	after	before	after	before	after
Breakfast						
Lunch						
Dinner						
Bedtime						

WEEK OF: __/__/__	SUNDAY		MONDAY		TUESDAY	
	before	after	before	after	before	after
Breakfast						
Lunch						
Dinner						
Bedtime						

WEEK OF: __/__/__	SUNDAY		MONDAY		TUESDAY	
	before	after	before	after	before	after
Breakfast						
Lunch						
Dinner						
Bedtime						

WEEK OF: __/__/__	SUNDAY		MONDAY		TUESDAY	
	before	after	before	after	before	after
Breakfast						
Lunch						
Dinner						
Bedtime						

BLOOD SUGAR LOG

Notes _____
_____
_____
_____

WEDNESDAY		THURSDAY		FRIDAY		SATURDAY	
before	after	before	after	before	after	before	after

WEDNESDAY		THURSDAY		FRIDAY		SATURDAY	
before	after	before	after	before	after	before	after

WEDNESDAY		THURSDAY		FRIDAY		SATURDAY	
before	after	before	after	before	after	before	after

WEDNESDAY		THURSDAY		FRIDAY		SATURDAY	
before	after	before	after	before	after	before	after

BLOOD SUGAR LOG

Notes _____

_____

_____

_____

WEEK OF: __/__/__	SUNDAY		MONDAY		TUESDAY	
	before	after	before	after	before	after
Breakfast						
Lunch						
Dinner						
Bedtime						

WEEK OF: __/__/__	SUNDAY		MONDAY		TUESDAY	
	before	after	before	after	before	after
Breakfast						
Lunch						
Dinner						
Bedtime						

WEEK OF: __/__/__	SUNDAY		MONDAY		TUESDAY	
	before	after	before	after	before	after
Breakfast						
Lunch						
Dinner						
Bedtime						

WEEK OF: __/__/__	SUNDAY		MONDAY		TUESDAY	
	before	after	before	after	before	after
Breakfast						
Lunch						
Dinner						
Bedtime						

BLOOD SUGAR LOG

Notes _____

_____

_____

_____

WEDNESDAY		THURSDAY		FRIDAY		SATURDAY	
before	after	before	after	before	after	before	after

WEDNESDAY		THURSDAY		FRIDAY		SATURDAY	
before	after	before	after	before	after	before	after

WEDNESDAY		THURSDAY		FRIDAY		SATURDAY	
before	after	before	after	before	after	before	after

WEDNESDAY		THURSDAY		FRIDAY		SATURDAY	
before	after	before	after	before	after	before	after

BLOOD SUGAR LOG

Notes _____

_____

_____

_____

WEEK OF: __/__/__	SUNDAY		MONDAY		TUESDAY	
	before	after	before	after	before	after
Breakfast						
Lunch						
Dinner						
Bedtime						

WEEK OF: __/__/__	SUNDAY		MONDAY		TUESDAY	
	before	after	before	after	before	after
Breakfast						
Lunch						
Dinner						
Bedtime						

WEEK OF: __/__/__	SUNDAY		MONDAY		TUESDAY	
	before	after	before	after	before	after
Breakfast						
Lunch						
Dinner						
Bedtime						

WEEK OF: __/__/__	SUNDAY		MONDAY		TUESDAY	
	before	after	before	after	before	after
Breakfast						
Lunch						
Dinner						
Bedtime						

BLOOD SUGAR LOG

Notes _____

_____

_____

_____

WEDNESDAY		THURSDAY		FRIDAY		SATURDAY	
before	after	before	after	before	after	before	after

WEDNESDAY		THURSDAY		FRIDAY		SATURDAY	
before	after	before	after	before	after	before	after

WEDNESDAY		THURSDAY		FRIDAY		SATURDAY	
before	after	before	after	before	after	before	after

WEDNESDAY		THURSDAY		FRIDAY		SATURDAY	
before	after	before	after	before	after	before	after

BLOOD SUGAR LOG

Notes _____

_____

_____

_____

WEEK OF: __/__/__	SUNDAY		MONDAY		TUESDAY	
	before	after	before	after	before	after
Breakfast						
Lunch						
Dinner						
Bedtime						

WEEK OF: __/__/__	SUNDAY		MONDAY		TUESDAY	
	before	after	before	after	before	after
Breakfast						
Lunch						
Dinner						
Bedtime						

WEEK OF: __/__/__	SUNDAY		MONDAY		TUESDAY	
	before	after	before	after	before	after
Breakfast						
Lunch						
Dinner						
Bedtime						

WEEK OF: __/__/__	SUNDAY		MONDAY		TUESDAY	
	before	after	before	after	before	after
Breakfast						
Lunch						
Dinner						
Bedtime						

BLOOD SUGAR LOG

Notes _____
_____
_____
_____

WEDNESDAY		THURSDAY		FRIDAY		SATURDAY	
before	after	before	after	before	after	before	after

WEDNESDAY		THURSDAY		FRIDAY		SATURDAY	
before	after	before	after	before	after	before	after

WEDNESDAY		THURSDAY		FRIDAY		SATURDAY	
before	after	before	after	before	after	before	after

WEDNESDAY		THURSDAY		FRIDAY		SATURDAY	
before	after	before	after	before	after	before	after

BLOOD SUGAR LOG

Notes _____
_____
_____
_____

WEEK OF: __/__/__	SUNDAY		MONDAY		TUESDAY	
	before	after	before	after	before	after
Breakfast						
Lunch						
Dinner						
Bedtime						

WEEK OF: __/__/__	SUNDAY		MONDAY		TUESDAY	
	before	after	before	after	before	after
Breakfast						
Lunch						
Dinner						
Bedtime						

WEEK OF: __/__/__	SUNDAY		MONDAY		TUESDAY	
	before	after	before	after	before	after
Breakfast						
Lunch						
Dinner						
Bedtime						

WEEK OF: __/__/__	SUNDAY		MONDAY		TUESDAY	
	before	after	before	after	before	after
Breakfast						
Lunch						
Dinner						
Bedtime						

BLOOD SUGAR LOG

Notes _____
_____
_____
_____

WEDNESDAY		THURSDAY		FRIDAY		SATURDAY	
before	after	before	after	before	after	before	after

WEDNESDAY		THURSDAY		FRIDAY		SATURDAY	
before	after	before	after	before	after	before	after

WEDNESDAY		THURSDAY		FRIDAY		SATURDAY	
before	after	before	after	before	after	before	after

WEDNESDAY		THURSDAY		FRIDAY		SATURDAY	
before	after	before	after	before	after	before	after

BLOOD SUGAR LOG

Notes _____

_____

_____

_____

WEEK OF: __/__/__	SUNDAY		MONDAY		TUESDAY	
	before	after	before	after	before	after
Breakfast						
Lunch						
Dinner						
Bedtime						

WEEK OF: __/__/__	SUNDAY		MONDAY		TUESDAY	
	before	after	before	after	before	after
Breakfast						
Lunch						
Dinner						
Bedtime						

WEEK OF: __/__/__	SUNDAY		MONDAY		TUESDAY	
	before	after	before	after	before	after
Breakfast						
Lunch						
Dinner						
Bedtime						

WEEK OF: __/__/__	SUNDAY		MONDAY		TUESDAY	
	before	after	before	after	before	after
Breakfast						
Lunch						
Dinner						
Bedtime						

BLOOD SUGAR LOG

Notes _____

_____

_____

_____

WEDNESDAY		THURSDAY		FRIDAY		SATURDAY	
before	after	before	after	before	after	before	after

WEDNESDAY		THURSDAY		FRIDAY		SATURDAY	
before	after	before	after	before	after	before	after

WEDNESDAY		THURSDAY		FRIDAY		SATURDAY	
before	after	before	after	before	after	before	after

WEDNESDAY		THURSDAY		FRIDAY		SATURDAY	
before	after	before	after	before	after	before	after

BLOOD SUGAR LOG

Notes _____
_____
_____
_____

WEEK OF: __/__/__	SUNDAY		MONDAY		TUESDAY	
	before	after	before	after	before	after
Breakfast						
Lunch						
Dinner						
Bedtime						

WEEK OF: __/__/__	SUNDAY		MONDAY		TUESDAY	
	before	after	before	after	before	after
Breakfast						
Lunch						
Dinner						
Bedtime						

WEEK OF: __/__/__	SUNDAY		MONDAY		TUESDAY	
	before	after	before	after	before	after
Breakfast						
Lunch						
Dinner						
Bedtime						

WEEK OF: __/__/__	SUNDAY		MONDAY		TUESDAY	
	before	after	before	after	before	after
Breakfast						
Lunch						
Dinner						
Bedtime						

BLOOD SUGAR LOG

Notes _____
_____
_____

WEDNESDAY		THURSDAY		FRIDAY		SATURDAY	
before	after	before	after	before	after	before	after

WEDNESDAY		THURSDAY		FRIDAY		SATURDAY	
before	after	before	after	before	after	before	after

WEDNESDAY		THURSDAY		FRIDAY		SATURDAY	
before	after	before	after	before	after	before	after

WEDNESDAY		THURSDAY		FRIDAY		SATURDAY	
before	after	before	after	before	after	before	after

BLOOD SUGAR LOG

Notes _____

_____

_____

WEEK OF: __/__/__	SUNDAY		MONDAY		TUESDAY	
	before	after	before	after	before	after
Breakfast						
Lunch						
Dinner						
Bedtime						

WEEK OF: __/__/__	SUNDAY		MONDAY		TUESDAY	
	before	after	before	after	before	after
Breakfast						
Lunch						
Dinner						
Bedtime						

WEEK OF: __/__/__	SUNDAY		MONDAY		TUESDAY	
	before	after	before	after	before	after
Breakfast						
Lunch						
Dinner						
Bedtime						

WEEK OF: __/__/__	SUNDAY		MONDAY		TUESDAY	
	before	after	before	after	before	after
Breakfast						
Lunch						
Dinner						
Bedtime						

BLOOD SUGAR LOG

Notes _____

_____

_____

_____

WEDNESDAY		THURSDAY		FRIDAY		SATURDAY	
before	after	before	after	before	after	before	after

WEDNESDAY		THURSDAY		FRIDAY		SATURDAY	
before	after	before	after	before	after	before	after

WEDNESDAY		THURSDAY		FRIDAY		SATURDAY	
before	after	before	after	before	after	before	after

WEDNESDAY		THURSDAY		FRIDAY		SATURDAY	
before	after	before	after	before	after	before	after

BLOOD SUGAR LOG

Notes _____

_____

_____

_____

WEEK OF: __/__/__	SUNDAY		MONDAY		TUESDAY	
	before	after	before	after	before	after
Breakfast						
Lunch						
Dinner						
Bedtime						

WEEK OF: __/__/__	SUNDAY		MONDAY		TUESDAY	
	before	after	before	after	before	after
Breakfast						
Lunch						
Dinner						
Bedtime						

WEEK OF: __/__/__	SUNDAY		MONDAY		TUESDAY	
	before	after	before	after	before	after
Breakfast						
Lunch						
Dinner						
Bedtime						

WEEK OF: __/__/__	SUNDAY		MONDAY		TUESDAY	
	before	after	before	after	before	after
Breakfast						
Lunch						
Dinner						
Bedtime						

BLOOD SUGAR LOG

Notes _____

_____

_____

_____

WEDNESDAY		THURSDAY		FRIDAY		SATURDAY	
before	after	before	after	before	after	before	after

WEDNESDAY		THURSDAY		FRIDAY		SATURDAY	
before	after	before	after	before	after	before	after

WEDNESDAY		THURSDAY		FRIDAY		SATURDAY	
before	after	before	after	before	after	before	after

WEDNESDAY		THURSDAY		FRIDAY		SATURDAY	
before	after	before	after	before	after	before	after

BLOOD SUGAR LOG

Notes _____

_____

_____

_____

WEEK OF: __/__/__	SUNDAY		MONDAY		TUESDAY	
	before	after	before	after	before	after
Breakfast						
Lunch						
Dinner						
Bedtime						

WEEK OF: __/__/__	SUNDAY		MONDAY		TUESDAY	
	before	after	before	after	before	after
Breakfast						
Lunch						
Dinner						
Bedtime						

WEEK OF: __/__/__	SUNDAY		MONDAY		TUESDAY	
	before	after	before	after	before	after
Breakfast						
Lunch						
Dinner						
Bedtime						

WEEK OF: __/__/__	SUNDAY		MONDAY		TUESDAY	
	before	after	before	after	before	after
Breakfast						
Lunch						
Dinner						
Bedtime						

BLOOD SUGAR LOG

Notes

WEDNESDAY		THURSDAY		FRIDAY		SATURDAY	
before	after	before	after	before	after	before	after

WEDNESDAY		THURSDAY		FRIDAY		SATURDAY	
before	after	before	after	before	after	before	after

WEDNESDAY		THURSDAY		FRIDAY		SATURDAY	
before	after	before	after	before	after	before	after

WEDNESDAY		THURSDAY		FRIDAY		SATURDAY	
before	after	before	after	before	after	before	after

BLOOD SUGAR LOG

Notes _____

_____

_____

WEEK OF: __/__/__	SUNDAY		MONDAY		TUESDAY	
	before	after	before	after	before	after
Breakfast						
Lunch						
Dinner						
Bedtime						

WEEK OF: __/__/__	SUNDAY		MONDAY		TUESDAY	
	before	after	before	after	before	after
Breakfast						
Lunch						
Dinner						
Bedtime						

WEEK OF: __/__/__	SUNDAY		MONDAY		TUESDAY	
	before	after	before	after	before	after
Breakfast						
Lunch						
Dinner						
Bedtime						

WEEK OF: __/__/__	SUNDAY		MONDAY		TUESDAY	
	before	after	before	after	before	after
Breakfast						
Lunch						
Dinner						
Bedtime						

BLOOD SUGAR LOG

Notes

WEDNESDAY		THURSDAY		FRIDAY		SATURDAY	
before	after	before	after	before	after	before	after

WEDNESDAY		THURSDAY		FRIDAY		SATURDAY	
before	after	before	after	before	after	before	after

WEDNESDAY		THURSDAY		FRIDAY		SATURDAY	
before	after	before	after	before	after	before	after

WEDNESDAY		THURSDAY		FRIDAY		SATURDAY	
before	after	before	after	before	after	before	after

BLOOD SUGAR LOG

Notes

WEEK OF: __/__/__	SUNDAY		MONDAY		TUESDAY	
	before	after	before	after	before	after
Breakfast						
Lunch						
Dinner						
Bedtime						

WEEK OF: __/__/__	SUNDAY		MONDAY		TUESDAY	
	before	after	before	after	before	after
Breakfast						
Lunch						
Dinner						
Bedtime						

WEEK OF: __/__/__	SUNDAY		MONDAY		TUESDAY	
	before	after	before	after	before	after
Breakfast						
Lunch						
Dinner						
Bedtime						

WEEK OF: __/__/__	SUNDAY		MONDAY		TUESDAY	
	before	after	before	after	before	after
Breakfast						
Lunch						
Dinner						
Bedtime						

BLOOD SUGAR LOG

Notes
_____
_____
_____
_____

WEDNESDAY		THURSDAY		FRIDAY		SATURDAY	
before	after	before	after	before	after	before	after

WEDNESDAY		THURSDAY		FRIDAY		SATURDAY	
before	after	before	after	before	after	before	after

WEDNESDAY		THURSDAY		FRIDAY		SATURDAY	
before	after	before	after	before	after	before	after

WEDNESDAY		THURSDAY		FRIDAY		SATURDAY	
before	after	before	after	before	after	before	after

BLOOD SUGAR LOG

Notes _____

_____

_____

_____

WEEK OF: __/__/__	SUNDAY		MONDAY		TUESDAY	
	before	after	before	after	before	after
Breakfast						
Lunch						
Dinner						
Bedtime						

WEEK OF: __/__/__	SUNDAY		MONDAY		TUESDAY	
	before	after	before	after	before	after
Breakfast						
Lunch						
Dinner						
Bedtime						

WEEK OF: __/__/__	SUNDAY		MONDAY		TUESDAY	
	before	after	before	after	before	after
Breakfast						
Lunch						
Dinner						
Bedtime						

WEEK OF: __/__/__	SUNDAY		MONDAY		TUESDAY	
	before	after	before	after	before	after
Breakfast						
Lunch						
Dinner						
Bedtime						

BLOOD SUGAR LOG

Notes _____

_____

_____

_____

WEDNESDAY		THURSDAY		FRIDAY		SATURDAY	
before	after	before	after	before	after	before	after

WEDNESDAY		THURSDAY		FRIDAY		SATURDAY	
before	after	before	after	before	after	before	after

WEDNESDAY		THURSDAY		FRIDAY		SATURDAY	
before	after	before	after	before	after	before	after

WEDNESDAY		THURSDAY		FRIDAY		SATURDAY	
before	after	before	after	before	after	before	after

BLOOD SUGAR LOG

Notes _____

_____

_____

_____

WEEK OF: __/__/__	SUNDAY		MONDAY		TUESDAY	
	before	after	before	after	before	after
Breakfast						
Lunch						
Dinner						
Bedtime						

WEEK OF: __/__/__	SUNDAY		MONDAY		TUESDAY	
	before	after	before	after	before	after
Breakfast						
Lunch						
Dinner						
Bedtime						

WEEK OF: __/__/__	SUNDAY		MONDAY		TUESDAY	
	before	after	before	after	before	after
Breakfast						
Lunch						
Dinner						
Bedtime						

WEEK OF: __/__/__	SUNDAY		MONDAY		TUESDAY	
	before	after	before	after	before	after
Breakfast						
Lunch						
Dinner						
Bedtime						

BLOOD SUGAR LOG

Notes _____

_____

_____

_____

WEDNESDAY		THURSDAY		FRIDAY		SATURDAY	
before	after	before	after	before	after	before	after

WEDNESDAY		THURSDAY		FRIDAY		SATURDAY	
before	after	before	after	before	after	before	after

WEDNESDAY		THURSDAY		FRIDAY		SATURDAY	
before	after	before	after	before	after	before	after

WEDNESDAY		THURSDAY		FRIDAY		SATURDAY	
before	after	before	after	before	after	before	after

BLOOD SUGAR LOG

Notes
_____
_____
_____
_____

WEEK OF: __/__/__	SUNDAY		MONDAY		TUESDAY	
	before	after	before	after	before	after
Breakfast						
Lunch						
Dinner						
Bedtime						

WEEK OF: __/__/__	SUNDAY		MONDAY		TUESDAY	
	before	after	before	after	before	after
Breakfast						
Lunch						
Dinner						
Bedtime						

WEEK OF: __/__/__	SUNDAY		MONDAY		TUESDAY	
	before	after	before	after	before	after
Breakfast						
Lunch						
Dinner						
Bedtime						

WEEK OF: __/__/__	SUNDAY		MONDAY		TUESDAY	
	before	after	before	after	before	after
Breakfast						
Lunch						
Dinner						
Bedtime						

BLOOD SUGAR LOG

Notes

WEDNESDAY		THURSDAY		FRIDAY		SATURDAY	
before	after	before	after	before	after	before	after

WEDNESDAY		THURSDAY		FRIDAY		SATURDAY	
before	after	before	after	before	after	before	after

WEDNESDAY		THURSDAY		FRIDAY		SATURDAY	
before	after	before	after	before	after	before	after

WEDNESDAY		THURSDAY		FRIDAY		SATURDAY	
before	after	before	after	before	after	before	after

BLOOD SUGAR LOG

Notes _____

_____

_____

_____

WEEK OF: __/__/__	SUNDAY		MONDAY		TUESDAY	
	before	after	before	after	before	after
Breakfast						
Lunch						
Dinner						
Bedtime						

WEEK OF: __/__/__	SUNDAY		MONDAY		TUESDAY	
	before	after	before	after	before	after
Breakfast						
Lunch						
Dinner						
Bedtime						

WEEK OF: __/__/__	SUNDAY		MONDAY		TUESDAY	
	before	after	before	after	before	after
Breakfast						
Lunch						
Dinner						
Bedtime						

WEEK OF: __/__/__	SUNDAY		MONDAY		TUESDAY	
	before	after	before	after	before	after
Breakfast						
Lunch						
Dinner						
Bedtime						

BLOOD SUGAR LOG

Notes _____
_____
_____
_____

WEDNESDAY		THURSDAY		FRIDAY		SATURDAY	
before	after	before	after	before	after	before	after

WEDNESDAY		THURSDAY		FRIDAY		SATURDAY	
before	after	before	after	before	after	before	after

WEDNESDAY		THURSDAY		FRIDAY		SATURDAY	
before	after	before	after	before	after	before	after

WEDNESDAY		THURSDAY		FRIDAY		SATURDAY	
before	after	before	after	before	after	before	after

BLOOD SUGAR LOG

Notes _____
_____
_____
_____

WEEK OF: __/__/__	SUNDAY		MONDAY		TUESDAY	
	before	after	before	after	before	after
Breakfast						
Lunch						
Dinner						
Bedtime						

WEEK OF: __/__/__	SUNDAY		MONDAY		TUESDAY	
	before	after	before	after	before	after
Breakfast						
Lunch						
Dinner						
Bedtime						

WEEK OF: __/__/__	SUNDAY		MONDAY		TUESDAY	
	before	after	before	after	before	after
Breakfast						
Lunch						
Dinner						
Bedtime						

WEEK OF: __/__/__	SUNDAY		MONDAY		TUESDAY	
	before	after	before	after	before	after
Breakfast						
Lunch						
Dinner						
Bedtime						

BLOOD SUGAR LOG

Notes _____

_____

_____

_____

WEDNESDAY		THURSDAY		FRIDAY		SATURDAY	
before	after	before	after	before	after	before	after

WEDNESDAY		THURSDAY		FRIDAY		SATURDAY	
before	after	before	after	before	after	before	after

WEDNESDAY		THURSDAY		FRIDAY		SATURDAY	
before	after	before	after	before	after	before	after

WEDNESDAY		THURSDAY		FRIDAY		SATURDAY	
before	after	before	after	before	after	before	after

BLOOD SUGAR LOG

Notes _____

_____

_____

_____

WEEK OF: __/__/__	SUNDAY		MONDAY		TUESDAY	
	before	after	before	after	before	after
Breakfast						
Lunch						
Dinner						
Bedtime						

WEEK OF: __/__/__	SUNDAY		MONDAY		TUESDAY	
	before	after	before	after	before	after
Breakfast						
Lunch						
Dinner						
Bedtime						

WEEK OF: __/__/__	SUNDAY		MONDAY		TUESDAY	
	before	after	before	after	before	after
Breakfast						
Lunch						
Dinner						
Bedtime						

WEEK OF: __/__/__	SUNDAY		MONDAY		TUESDAY	
	before	after	before	after	before	after
Breakfast						
Lunch						
Dinner						
Bedtime						

BLOOD SUGAR LOG

Notes _____

_____

_____

_____

WEDNESDAY		THURSDAY		FRIDAY		SATURDAY	
before	after	before	after	before	after	before	after

WEDNESDAY		THURSDAY		FRIDAY		SATURDAY	
before	after	before	after	before	after	before	after

WEDNESDAY		THURSDAY		FRIDAY		SATURDAY	
before	after	before	after	before	after	before	after

WEDNESDAY		THURSDAY		FRIDAY		SATURDAY	
before	after	before	after	before	after	before	after

BLOOD SUGAR LOG

Notes _____

_____

_____

_____

WEEK OF: __/__/__	SUNDAY		MONDAY		TUESDAY	
	before	after	before	after	before	after
Breakfast						
Lunch						
Dinner						
Bedtime						

WEEK OF: __/__/__	SUNDAY		MONDAY		TUESDAY	
	before	after	before	after	before	after
Breakfast						
Lunch						
Dinner						
Bedtime						

WEEK OF: __/__/__	SUNDAY		MONDAY		TUESDAY	
	before	after	before	after	before	after
Breakfast						
Lunch						
Dinner						
Bedtime						

WEEK OF: __/__/__	SUNDAY		MONDAY		TUESDAY	
	before	after	before	after	before	after
Breakfast						
Lunch						
Dinner						
Bedtime						

BLOOD SUGAR LOG

Notes

WEDNESDAY		THURSDAY		FRIDAY		SATURDAY	
before	after	before	after	before	after	before	after

WEDNESDAY		THURSDAY		FRIDAY		SATURDAY	
before	after	before	after	before	after	before	after

WEDNESDAY		THURSDAY		FRIDAY		SATURDAY	
before	after	before	after	before	after	before	after

WEDNESDAY		THURSDAY		FRIDAY		SATURDAY	
before	after	before	after	before	after	before	after

BLOOD SUGAR LOG

Notes _____
_____
_____
_____

WEEK OF: __/__/__	SUNDAY		MONDAY		TUESDAY	
	before	after	before	after	before	after
Breakfast						
Lunch						
Dinner						
Bedtime						

WEEK OF: __/__/__	SUNDAY		MONDAY		TUESDAY	
	before	after	before	after	before	after
Breakfast						
Lunch						
Dinner						
Bedtime						

WEEK OF: __/__/__	SUNDAY		MONDAY		TUESDAY	
	before	after	before	after	before	after
Breakfast						
Lunch						
Dinner						
Bedtime						

WEEK OF: __/__/__	SUNDAY		MONDAY		TUESDAY	
	before	after	before	after	before	after
Breakfast						
Lunch						
Dinner						
Bedtime